THE
WELL JOURNAL

Eat Well, Live Well

Mia Rigden

CLARKSON POTTER/PUBLISHERS

New York

"ONE CANNOT

THINK WELL,

LOVE WELL,

SLEEP WELL,

IF ONE HAS NOT

DINED WELL."

—VIRGINIA WOOLF

WELCOME TO *THE WELL JOURNAL.*

This bite-size book was born out of extensive research and experience watching people's lives change as they altered their eating habits. As a nutritionist, I've seen countless pounds and inches lost, but the most remarkable shifts are never reflected on the scale. Some of the most profound benefits of adopting healthy habits include increased energy, mood, and productivity, improved sleep, stronger relationships, and finding joy in eating nutrient-dense foods.

Diets don't work because they don't fit into our lives. They generally have a start and an end date, involve restrictive or labor-intensive meals (which you probably don't enjoy), and are very difficult to sustain while traveling, celebrating birthdays, at work events—or basically, just living a real life! Instead of looking toward fad diets, trendy supplements, or magical potions to answer your wellness woes, focus on creating healthy lifestyle habits.[1] Incorporating even the smallest changes can make a big impact over time, and when you discover foods that make you feel as great as they taste, you'll never have to diet again.

So how do you get there? The only way to change your actions is to be aware of them in the first place. Studies consistently show that self-monitoring leads to positive health outcomes,[2] including weight loss,[3,4] increased physical activity levels, and overall consciousness of both quantity and quality of foods consumed.

This journal is not about counting calories—in fact, I wholeheartedly discourage it. Completing your daily entries is really an exercise in mindfulness. Whether you constantly snack at work, overindulge in sweets after dinner, or generally don't eat enough vegetables, your journal will help you recognize these habits, the conditions in which they take place, and their long- and short-term effects.

While what you eat is undeniably important, when it comes to changing habits, it's critical to also take note of the why and the how. Where are you hitting roadblocks? What are the situations and circumstances that prevent you from making the healthy choices that you want to make? How can you learn from all those times you've felt tired, irritable, bloated, or unwell, and how can you make food choices that will support the lifestyle and person you aspire to be?

There is not one way of eating that works for everyone. We are all unique and magical beings; like different foods; were brought up differently; have distinct genetics and biology; have different work schedules, family and social obligations; and have cultural and religious practices that influence what we eat.

It is my hope that the following pages will help you connect the dots. How do your eating habits support (or hinder) your quality of life? Nutrition is not an isolated part of your world. It is deeply connected to every part of you—physically, mentally, and spiritually. When you take the time to truly understand your body and your lifestyle, you will know exactly how you need to nourish it.

There is no right or wrong way to fill out your journal entries, but I do have one important rule: no judgments! Certain occasions call for indulgences and that's okay. These journals are not meant to be perfect, they're meant to be real. This is powerful information that you can use to achieve your wellness, personal, and professional goals.

Celebrate your best days and learn from the challenging ones. Use these pages to empower yourself to find wonderfully delicious and satisfying foods that make you look and feel your very best.

X

MIA RIGDEN
Nutritionist & Founder, RASA

A LITTLE NUTRITION ADVICE

While everyone is different, we could all benefit from a few basic dietary principles. Here are my top ten. Keep these in mind when completing and assessing your journal entries.

DELICIOUS FIRST.

Life is too short to eat food you don't love. If your "healthy" meals are not also super tasty, you won't be eating them for long.

EAT YOUR VEGGIES!

Make vegetables the star of your plate. Aim not just for five to seven servings of vegetables a day but also for diversity. The greater variety of vegetables you consume, the more nutrients you're getting! See if you can consume twenty different vegetables per week.

FOCUS ON QUALITY OVER QUANTITY.

Instead of counting calories, place an emphasis on quality whole foods. Buy organic whenever possible. When it comes to animal protein, choose organic, pasture-raised eggs and poultry, all-grass-fed meat and wild seafood.

READ LABELS.

If you're not already in the habit of flipping over every jar of peanut butter and carton of nut milk, get into it. Look out for excessive sugar, processed oils, and unfamiliar ingredients. And don't be fooled by terms like *gluten free*, *organic*, or *all natural*. Food marketers are often one step ahead of us.

ELIMINATE PROCESSED FOODS AND EXCESS SUGAR.

Reduce your intake of processed foods containing inflammatory vegetable oils (canola, soy, sunflower, etc.) and sugar. As a rule of thumb, avoid anything packaged with more than 10g of sugar per serving.

DRINK WATER.

This tried-and-true tip lives up to every bit of the hype. The daily recommended amount of water is half your body weight in ounces. You can do it. Gulp gulp.

PRIORITIZE SLEEP!

Rest is incredibly important for all our bodily systems, including digestion, immunity, cellular repair, cognitive function, and more. Plus, your hunger hormones are regulated in part by your sleeping patterns. Less sleep equals more hunger.

BE PREPARED.

Think about your day and plan your meals in advance, so you can set yourself up for success. Look out for patterns in your journal entries—like coming home from work starving or that 4pm trip to the candy drawer—and try to find solutions.

STAY POSITIVE.

Your gut and your brain are partners in this game. Find your practice: yoga, meditation, snuggles, painting, hiking, etc. Whatever makes you happy, do more of that.

DON'T STRESS.

No one is perfect. What you eat the majority of the time will have a larger impact on your health than the random cheese and cracker indulgence. And stress is counterproductive—it messes with your hormones, digestion, mental health, and so much more.

COMMITMENT

I, ———————————————— , commit to consistently writing in my Well Journal and will reflect upon my entries not with judgment but from a place of love and understanding.

———————————————————————

SIGNATURE

———————————————————————

DATE

———

GOALS

Use these pages to document your dreams, whether big, small, or somewhere in between, and come up with actionable steps to make them a reality. These goals do not need to be food or wellness related. They certainly can be, but feel free to log your deepest and wildest aspirations here. Go get 'em!

GOAL 1

_____

_____

_____

List five actionable steps to get there:

1. _____

2. _____

3. _____

4. _____

5. _____

GOAL 2

_____

_____

_____

List five actionable steps to get there:

1. _____

2. _____

3. _____

4. _____

5. _____

GOAL 3

_____

_____

_____

List five actionable steps to get there:

1. _____

2. _____

3. _____

4. _____

5. _____

GOAL 4

_____

_____

_____

List five actionable steps to get there:

1. _____

2. _____

3. _____

4. _____

5. _____

DATE: / /

How are you feeling today?

UGH   OK   GOOD   AWESOME

How did you sleep last night?

_____

Breakfast   TIME: _____

FOOD: _____

_____

_____

DRINKS: _____

Lunch   TIME: _____

FOOD: _____

_____

_____

DRINKS: _____

Dinner   TIME: _____

FOOD: _____

_____

_____

DRINKS: _____

Snacks/Other   TIME(S): _____

_____

_____

Supplements/Medications (if applicable)

_____

How many servings of vegetables did you eat today? ——————————

Exercise

_____

Mindfulness practice

_____

List three things you are grateful for:

1. _____

2. _____

3. _____

What went well today?

_____

_____

_____

LET IT OUT

_____

_____

_____

_____

_____

How are you feeling today?

UGH   OK   GOOD   AWESOME

How did you sleep last night?

_____

Breakfast   TIME: _____

FOOD: _____

_____

_____

DRINKS: _____

Lunch   TIME: _____

FOOD: _____

_____

_____

DRINKS: _____

Dinner   TIME: _____

FOOD: _____

_____

_____

DRINKS: _____

Snacks/Other   TIME(S): _____

_____

_____

Supplements/Medications (if applicable)

_____

How many servings of vegetables did you eat today? _____

Exercise

_____

Mindfulness practice

_____

List three things you are grateful for:

1. _____

2. _____

3. _____

What went well today?

_____

_____

_____

LET IT OUT

_____

_____

_____

_____

_____

DATE: /   /

How are you feeling today?

UGH   OK   GOOD   AWESOME

How did you sleep last night?

_____

Breakfast   TIME: _____

FOOD: _____

_____

_____

DRINKS: _____

Lunch   TIME: _____

FOOD: _____

_____

_____

DRINKS: _____

Dinner   TIME: _____

FOOD: _____

_____

_____

DRINKS: _____

Snacks/Other   TIME(S): _____

_____

_____

Supplements/Medications (if applicable)

_____

How many servings of vegetables did you eat today? ——————————

Exercise

_____

Mindfulness practice

_____

List three things you are grateful for:

1. _____

2. _____

3. _____

What went well today?

_____

_____

_____

LET IT OUT

_____

_____

_____

_____

_____

DATE: / /

How are you feeling today?

UGH   OK   GOOD   AWESOME

How did you sleep last night?

_____

Breakfast   TIME: _____

FOOD: _____

_____

_____

DRINKS: _____

Lunch   TIME: _____

FOOD: _____

_____

_____

DRINKS: _____

Dinner   TIME: _____

FOOD: _____

_____

_____

DRINKS: _____

Snacks/Other   TIME(S): _____

_____

_____

Supplements/Medications (if applicable)

_____

How many servings of vegetables did you eat today? _____

Exercise

_____

Mindfulness practice

_____

List three things you are grateful for:

1. _____

2. _____

3. _____

What went well today?

_____

_____

_____

LET IT OUT

_____

_____

_____

_____

_____

DATE: /   /

How are you feeling today?

UGH   OK   GOOD   AWESOME

How did you sleep last night?

_____

Breakfast   TIME: _____

FOOD: _____

_____

_____

DRINKS: _____

Lunch   TIME: _____

FOOD: _____

_____

_____

DRINKS: _____

Dinner   TIME: _____

FOOD: _____

_____

_____

DRINKS: _____

Snacks/Other   TIME(S): _____

_____

_____

Supplements/Medications (if applicable)

_____

How many servings of vegetables did you eat today? ———————————

Exercise

_____

Mindfulness practice

_____

List three things you are grateful for:

1. _____

2. _____

3. _____

What went well today?

_____

_____

_____

LET IT OUT

_____

_____

_____

_____

_____

DATE: / /

How are you feeling today?

UGH   OK   GOOD   AWESOME

How did you sleep last night?

_____

Breakfast   TIME: _____

FOOD: _____

_____

_____

DRINKS: _____

Lunch   TIME: _____

FOOD: _____

_____

_____

DRINKS: _____

Dinner   TIME: _____

FOOD: _____

_____

_____

DRINKS: _____

Snacks/Other   TIME(S): _____

_____

_____

Supplements/Medications (if applicable)

_____

How many servings of vegetables did you eat today? _____

Exercise

_____

Mindfulness practice

_____

List three things you are grateful for:

1. _____
2. _____
3. _____

What went well today?

_____

_____

_____

LET IT OUT

_____

_____

_____

_____

_____

DATE: / /

How are you feeling today?

UGH   OK   GOOD   AWESOME

How did you sleep last night?

_____

Breakfast   TIME: _____

FOOD: _____

_____

_____

DRINKS: _____

Lunch   TIME: _____

FOOD: _____

_____

_____

DRINKS: _____

Dinner   TIME: _____

FOOD: _____

_____

_____

DRINKS: _____

Snacks/Other   TIME(S): _____

_____

_____

Supplements/Medications (if applicable)

_____

How many servings of vegetables did you eat today? _____

Exercise

_____

Mindfulness practice

_____

List three things you are grateful for:

1. _____
2. _____
3. _____

What went well today?

_____
_____
_____

LET IT OUT

_____
_____
_____
_____
_____

DATE: /   /

How are you feeling today?

UGH   OK   GOOD   AWESOME

How did you sleep last night?

_____

Breakfast   TIME: _____

FOOD: _____

_____

_____

DRINKS: _____

Lunch   TIME: _____

FOOD: _____

_____

_____

DRINKS: _____

Dinner   TIME: _____

FOOD: _____

_____

_____

DRINKS: _____

Snacks/Other   TIME(S): _____

_____

_____

Supplements/Medications (if applicable)

_____

How many servings of vegetables did you eat today? _____

Exercise

_____

Mindfulness practice

_____

List three things you are grateful for:

1. _____

2. _____

3. _____

What went well today?

_____

_____

_____

LET IT OUT

_____

_____

_____

_____

_____

DATE: /   /

How are you feeling today?

UGH   OK   GOOD   AWESOME

How did you sleep last night?

_____

Breakfast   TIME: _____

FOOD: _____

_____

_____

DRINKS: _____

Lunch   TIME: _____

FOOD: _____

_____

_____

DRINKS: _____

Dinner   TIME: _____

FOOD: _____

_____

_____

DRINKS: _____

Snacks/Other   TIME(S): _____

_____

_____

Supplements/Medications (if applicable)

_____

How many servings of vegetables did you eat today? _____

Exercise

_____

Mindfulness practice

_____

List three things you are grateful for:

1. _____

2. _____

3. _____

What went well today?

_____

_____

_____

LET IT OUT

_____

_____

_____

_____

_____

DATE: / /

How are you feeling today?

UGH   OK   GOOD   AWESOME

How did you sleep last night?

_____

Breakfast   TIME: _____

FOOD: _____

_____

_____

DRINKS: _____

Lunch   TIME: _____

FOOD: _____

_____

_____

DRINKS: _____

Dinner   TIME: _____

FOOD: _____

_____

_____

DRINKS: _____

Snacks/Other   TIME(S): _____

_____

_____

Supplements/Medications (if applicable)

_____

How many servings of vegetables did you eat today? ——————————

Exercise

_____

Mindfulness practice

_____

List three things you are grateful for:

1. _____

2. _____

3. _____

What went well today?

_____

_____

_____

LET IT OUT

_____

_____

_____

_____

DATE: / /

How are you feeling today?

UGH   OK   GOOD   AWESOME

How did you sleep last night?

_____

Breakfast   TIME: _____

FOOD: _____

_____

_____

DRINKS: _____

Lunch   TIME: _____

FOOD: _____

_____

_____

DRINKS: _____

Dinner   TIME: _____

FOOD: _____

_____

_____

DRINKS: _____

Snacks/Other   TIME(S): _____

_____

_____

Supplements/Medications (if applicable)

_____

How many servings of vegetables did you eat today? _____

Exercise

_____

Mindfulness practice

_____

List three things you are grateful for:

1. _____

2. _____

3. _____

What went well today?

_____

_____

_____

LET IT OUT

_____

_____

_____

_____

_____

DATE: / /

How are you feeling today?

UGH   OK   GOOD   AWESOME

How did you sleep last night?

_____

Breakfast   TIME: _____

FOOD: _____
_____
_____

DRINKS: _____

Lunch   TIME: _____

FOOD: _____
_____
_____

DRINKS: _____

Dinner   TIME: _____

FOOD: _____
_____
_____

DRINKS: _____

Snacks/Other   TIME(S): _____

_____
_____

Supplements/Medications (if applicable)

_____

How many servings of vegetables did you eat today? _____

Exercise

_____

Mindfulness practice

_____

List three things you are grateful for:

1. _____

2. _____

3. _____

What went well today?

_____

_____

_____

LET IT OUT

_____

_____

_____

_____

_____

DATE: /   /

How are you feeling today?

UGH   OK   GOOD   AWESOME

How did you sleep last night?

_____

Breakfast   TIME: _____

FOOD: _____

_____

_____

DRINKS: _____

Lunch   TIME: _____

FOOD: _____

_____

_____

DRINKS: _____

Dinner   TIME: _____

FOOD: _____

_____

_____

DRINKS: _____

Snacks/Other   TIME(S): _____

_____

_____

Supplements/Medications (if applicable)

How many servings of vegetables did you eat today? ————————

Exercise

Mindfulness practice

List three things you are grateful for:

1.

2.

3.

What went well today?

LET IT OUT

DATE: / /

How are you feeling today?

UGH   OK   GOOD   AWESOME

How did you sleep last night?

_____

Breakfast   TIME: _____

FOOD: _____

_____

_____

DRINKS: _____

Lunch   TIME: _____

FOOD: _____

_____

_____

DRINKS: _____

Dinner   TIME: _____

FOOD: _____

_____

_____

DRINKS: _____

Snacks/Other   TIME(S): _____

_____

_____

Supplements/Medications (if applicable)

_____

How many servings of vegetables did you eat today? _____

Exercise

_____

Mindfulness practice

_____

List three things you are grateful for:

1. _____

2. _____

3. _____

What went well today?

_____

_____

_____

LET IT OUT

_____

_____

_____

_____

_____

DATE: /   /

How are you feeling today?

UGH   OK   GOOD   AWESOME

How did you sleep last night?

_____

Breakfast   TIME: _____

FOOD: _____

_____

_____

DRINKS: _____

Lunch   TIME: _____

FOOD: _____

_____

_____

DRINKS: _____

Dinner   TIME: _____

FOOD: _____

_____

_____

DRINKS: _____

Snacks/Other   TIME(S): _____

_____

_____

Supplements/Medications (if applicable)

_____

How many servings of vegetables did you eat today? _____

Exercise

_____

Mindfulness practice

_____

List three things you are grateful for:

1. _____

2. _____

3. _____

What went well today?

_____

_____

_____

LET IT OUT

_____

_____

_____

_____

_____

How are you feeling today?

UGH   OK   GOOD   AWESOME

How did you sleep last night?

_____

Breakfast   TIME: _____

FOOD: _____

_____

_____

DRINKS: _____

Lunch   TIME: _____

FOOD: _____

_____

_____

DRINKS: _____

Dinner   TIME: _____

FOOD: _____

_____

_____

DRINKS: _____

Snacks/Other   TIME(S): _____

_____

_____

Supplements/Medications (if applicable)

_____

How many servings of vegetables did you eat today? _____

Exercise

_____

Mindfulness practice

_____

List three things you are grateful for:

1. _____

2. _____

3. _____

What went well today?

_____

_____

_____

LET IT OUT

_____

_____

_____

_____

_____

DATE: / /

How are you feeling today?

UGH   OK   GOOD   AWESOME

How did you sleep last night?

_____

Breakfast   TIME: _____

FOOD: _____

_____

_____

DRINKS: _____

Lunch   TIME: _____

FOOD: _____

_____

_____

DRINKS: _____

Dinner   TIME: _____

FOOD: _____

_____

_____

DRINKS: _____

Snacks/Other   TIME(S): _____

_____

_____

Supplements/Medications (if applicable)

_____

How many servings of vegetables did you eat today? _____

Exercise

_____

Mindfulness practice

_____

List three things you are grateful for:

1. _____

2. _____

3. _____

What went well today?

_____

_____

_____

LET IT OUT

_____

_____

_____

_____

_____

DATE: / /

How are you feeling today?

UGH   OK   GOOD   AWESOME

How did you sleep last night?

_____

Breakfast   TIME: _____

FOOD: _____

_____

_____

DRINKS: _____

Lunch   TIME: _____

FOOD: _____

_____

_____

DRINKS: _____

Dinner   TIME: _____

FOOD: _____

_____

_____

DRINKS: _____

Snacks/Other   TIME(S): _____

_____

_____

Supplements/Medications (if applicable)

_____

How many servings of vegetables did you eat today? _____

Exercise

_____

Mindfulness practice

_____

List three things you are grateful for:

1. _____

2. _____

3. _____

What went well today?

_____

_____

_____

LET IT OUT

_____

_____

_____

_____

_____

DATE: /   /

How are you feeling today?

UGH   OK   GOOD   AWESOME

How did you sleep last night?

_____

Breakfast   TIME: _____

FOOD: _____

_____

_____

DRINKS: _____

Lunch   TIME: _____

FOOD: _____

_____

_____

DRINKS: _____

Dinner   TIME: _____

FOOD: _____

_____

_____

DRINKS: _____

Snacks/Other   TIME(S): _____

_____

_____

Supplements/Medications (if applicable)

_____

How many servings of vegetables did you eat today? _____

Exercise

_____

Mindfulness practice

_____

List three things you are grateful for:

1. _____

2. _____

3. _____

What went well today?

_____

_____

_____

LET IT OUT

_____

_____

_____

_____

_____

DATE: /   /

How are you feeling today?

UGH   OK   GOOD   AWESOME

How did you sleep last night?

_____

Breakfast   TIME: _____

FOOD: _____

_____

_____

DRINKS: _____

Lunch   TIME: _____

FOOD: _____

_____

_____

DRINKS: _____

Dinner   TIME: _____

FOOD: _____

_____

_____

DRINKS: _____

Snacks/Other   TIME(S): _____

_____

_____

Supplements/Medications (if applicable)

_____

How many servings of vegetables did you eat today? _____

Exercise

_____

Mindfulness practice

_____

List three things you are grateful for:

1. _____

2. _____

3. _____

What went well today?

_____

_____

_____

LET IT OUT

_____

_____

_____

_____

_____

DATE: / /

How are you feeling today?

UGH   OK   GOOD   AWESOME

How did you sleep last night?

_____

Breakfast   TIME: _____

FOOD: _____

_____

_____

DRINKS: _____

Lunch   TIME: _____

FOOD: _____

_____

_____

DRINKS: _____

Dinner   TIME: _____

FOOD: _____

_____

_____

DRINKS: _____

Snacks/Other   TIME(S): _____

_____

_____

Supplements/Medications (if applicable)

_____

How many servings of vegetables did you eat today? _____

Exercise

_____

Mindfulness practice

_____

List three things you are grateful for:

1. _____

2. _____

3. _____

What went well today?

_____

_____

_____

LET IT OUT

_____

_____

_____

_____

_____

DATE: / /

How are you feeling today?

UGH   OK   GOOD   AWESOME

How did you sleep last night?

_____

Breakfast   TIME: _____

FOOD: _____

_____

_____

DRINKS: _____

Lunch   TIME: _____

FOOD: _____

_____

_____

DRINKS: _____

Dinner   TIME: _____

FOOD: _____

_____

_____

DRINKS: _____

Snacks/Other   TIME(S): _____

_____

_____

Supplements/Medications (if applicable)

_____

How many servings of vegetables did you eat today? _____

Exercise

_____

Mindfulness practice

_____

List three things you are grateful for:

1. _____

2. _____

3. _____

What went well today?

_____

_____

_____

LET IT OUT

_____

_____

_____

_____

_____

DATE: / /

How are you feeling today?

UGH   OK   GOOD   AWESOME

How did you sleep last night?

_____

Breakfast   TIME:

FOOD:
_____

_____

_____

DRINKS:
_____

Lunch   TIME:

FOOD:
_____

_____

_____

DRINKS:
_____

Dinner   TIME:

FOOD:
_____

_____

_____

DRINKS:
_____

Snacks/Other   TIME(S):

_____

_____

Supplements/Medications (if applicable)

_____

How many servings of vegetables did you eat today? _____

Exercise

_____

Mindfulness practice

_____

List three things you are grateful for:

1. _____

2. _____

3. _____

What went well today?

_____

_____

_____

LET IT OUT

_____

_____

_____

_____

_____

DATE: /   /

How are you feeling today?

UGH   OK   GOOD   AWESOME

How did you sleep last night?

_____

Breakfast   TIME: _____

FOOD: _____

_____

_____

DRINKS: _____

Lunch   TIME: _____

FOOD: _____

_____

_____

DRINKS: _____

Dinner   TIME: _____

FOOD: _____

_____

_____

DRINKS: _____

Snacks/Other   TIME(S): _____

_____

_____

Supplements/Medications (if applicable)

_____

How many servings of vegetables did you eat today? ——————————

Exercise

_____

Mindfulness practice

_____

List three things you are grateful for:

1. _____

2. _____

3. _____

What went well today?

_____

_____

_____

LET IT OUT

_____

_____

_____

_____

_____

DATE: / /

How are you feeling today?

UGH   OK   GOOD   AWESOME

How did you sleep last night?

_____

Breakfast   TIME: _____

FOOD: _____

_____

_____

DRINKS: _____

Lunch   TIME: _____

FOOD: _____

_____

_____

DRINKS: _____

Dinner   TIME: _____

FOOD: _____

_____

_____

DRINKS: _____

Snacks/Other   TIME(S): _____

_____

_____

Supplements/Medications (if applicable)

_____

How many servings of vegetables did you eat today? _____

Exercise

_____

Mindfulness practice

_____

List three things you are grateful for:

1. _____

2. _____

3. _____

What went well today?

_____

_____

_____

LET IT OUT

_____

_____

_____

_____

_____

DATE: /   /

How are you feeling today?

UGH   OK   GOOD   AWESOME

How did you sleep last night?

_____

Breakfast   TIME: _____

FOOD: _____

_____

_____

DRINKS: _____

Lunch   TIME: _____

FOOD: _____

_____

_____

DRINKS: _____

Dinner   TIME: _____

FOOD: _____

_____

_____

DRINKS: _____

Snacks/Other   TIME(S): _____

_____

_____

Supplements/Medications (if applicable)

_____

How many servings of vegetables did you eat today? _____

Exercise

_____

Mindfulness practice

_____

List three things you are grateful for:

1. _____

2. _____

3. _____

What went well today?

_____

_____

_____

LET IT OUT

_____

_____

_____

_____

_____

DATE: / /

How are you feeling today?

UGH   OK   GOOD   AWESOME

How did you sleep last night?

_____

Breakfast   TIME: _____

FOOD: _____

_____

_____

DRINKS: _____

Lunch   TIME: _____

FOOD: _____

_____

_____

DRINKS: _____

Dinner   TIME: _____

FOOD: _____

_____

_____

DRINKS: _____

Snacks/Other   TIME(S): _____

_____

_____

Supplements/Medications (if applicable)

How many servings of vegetables did you eat today? ————————————

Exercise

Mindfulness practice

List three things you are grateful for:

1.

2.

3.

What went well today?

LET IT OUT

DATE: /   /

How are you feeling today?

UGH   OK   GOOD   AWESOME

How did you sleep last night?

_____

Breakfast   TIME: _____

FOOD: _____

_____

_____

DRINKS: _____

Lunch   TIME: _____

FOOD: _____

_____

_____

DRINKS: _____

Dinner   TIME: _____

FOOD: _____

_____

_____

DRINKS: _____

Snacks/Other   TIME(S): _____

_____

_____

Supplements/Medications (if applicable)

_____

How many servings of vegetables did you eat today? _____

Exercise

_____

Mindfulness practice

_____

List three things you are grateful for:

1. _____

2. _____

3. _____

What went well today?

_____

_____

_____

LET IT OUT

_____

_____

_____

_____

_____

DATE: / /

How are you feeling today?

UGH   OK   GOOD   AWESOME

How did you sleep last night?

_____

Breakfast   TIME: _____

FOOD: _____

_____

_____

DRINKS: _____

Lunch   TIME: _____

FOOD: _____

_____

_____

DRINKS: _____

Dinner   TIME: _____

FOOD: _____

_____

_____

DRINKS: _____

Snacks/Other   TIME(S): _____

_____

_____

Supplements/Medications (if applicable)

_____

How many servings of vegetables did you eat today? —————————————

Exercise

_____

Mindfulness practice

_____

List three things you are grateful for:

1. _____

2. _____

3. _____

What went well today?

_____

_____

_____

LET IT OUT

_____

_____

_____

_____

_____

DATE: /   /

How are you feeling today?

UGH   OK   GOOD   AWESOME

How did you sleep last night?

_____

Breakfast   TIME: _____

FOOD: _____

_____

_____

DRINKS: _____

Lunch   TIME: _____

FOOD: _____

_____

_____

DRINKS: _____

Dinner   TIME: _____

FOOD: _____

_____

_____

DRINKS: _____

Snacks/Other   TIME(S): _____

_____

_____

Supplements/Medications (if applicable)

_____

How many servings of vegetables did you eat today? _____

Exercise

_____

Mindfulness practice

_____

List three things you are grateful for:

1. _____

2. _____

3. _____

What went well today?

_____

_____

_____

LET IT OUT

_____

_____

_____

_____

_____

DATE: /   /

How are you feeling today?

UGH   OK   GOOD   AWESOME

How did you sleep last night?

_____

Breakfast   TIME: _____

FOOD: _____

_____

_____

DRINKS: _____

Lunch   TIME: _____

FOOD: _____

_____

_____

DRINKS: _____

Dinner   TIME: _____

FOOD: _____

_____

_____

DRINKS: _____

Snacks/Other   TIME(S): _____

_____

_____

Supplements/Medications (if applicable)

_____

How many servings of vegetables did you eat today? _____

Exercise

_____

Mindfulness practice

_____

List three things you are grateful for:

1. _____

2. _____

3. _____

What went well today?

_____

_____

_____

LET IT OUT

_____

_____

_____

_____

_____

DATE: / /

How are you feeling today?

UGH   OK   GOOD   AWESOME

How did you sleep last night?

_____

Breakfast   TIME: _____

FOOD: _____

_____

_____

DRINKS: _____

Lunch   TIME: _____

FOOD: _____

_____

_____

DRINKS: _____

Dinner   TIME: _____

FOOD: _____

_____

_____

DRINKS: _____

Snacks/Other   TIME(S): _____

_____

_____

Supplements/Medications (if applicable)

_____

How many servings of vegetables did you eat today? _____

Exercise

_____

Mindfulness practice

_____

List three things you are grateful for:

1. _____

2. _____

3. _____

What went well today?

_____

_____

_____

LET IT OUT

_____

_____

_____

_____

_____

DATE: / /

How are you feeling today?

UGH   OK   GOOD   AWESOME

How did you sleep last night?

_____

Breakfast   TIME: _____

FOOD: _____

_____

_____

DRINKS: _____

Lunch   TIME: _____

FOOD: _____

_____

_____

DRINKS: _____

Dinner   TIME: _____

FOOD: _____

_____

_____

DRINKS: _____

Snacks/Other   TIME(S): _____

_____

_____

Supplements/Medications (if applicable)

_____

How many servings of vegetables did you eat today? _____

Exercise

_____

Mindfulness practice

_____

List three things you are grateful for:

1. _____

2. _____

3. _____

What went well today?

_____

_____

_____

LET IT OUT

_____

_____

_____

_____

_____

DATE: / /

How are you feeling today?

UGH   OK   GOOD   AWESOME

How did you sleep last night?

_____

Breakfast   TIME: _____

FOOD: _____

_____

_____

DRINKS: _____

Lunch   TIME: _____

FOOD: _____

_____

_____

DRINKS: _____

Dinner   TIME: _____

FOOD: _____

_____

_____

DRINKS: _____

Snacks/Other   TIME(S): _____

_____

_____

Supplements/Medications (if applicable)

_____

How many servings of vegetables did you eat today? _____

Exercise

_____

Mindfulness practice

_____

List three things you are grateful for:

1. _____

2. _____

3. _____

What went well today?

_____

_____

_____

LET IT OUT

_____

_____

_____

_____

DATE: / /

How are you feeling today?

UGH   OK   GOOD   AWESOME

How did you sleep last night?

_____

Breakfast   TIME: _____

FOOD: _____

_____

_____

DRINKS: _____

Lunch   TIME: _____

FOOD: _____

_____

_____

DRINKS: _____

Dinner   TIME: _____

FOOD: _____

_____

_____

DRINKS: _____

Snacks/Other   TIME(S): _____

_____

_____

Supplements/Medications (if applicable)

_____

How many servings of vegetables did you eat today? _____

Exercise

_____

Mindfulness practice

_____

List three things you are grateful for:

1. _____

2. _____

3. _____

What went well today?

_____

_____

_____

LET IT OUT

_____

_____

_____

_____

_____

DATE: / /

How are you feeling today?

UGH   OK   GOOD   AWESOME

How did you sleep last night?

_____

Breakfast   TIME: _____

FOOD: _____

_____

_____

DRINKS: _____

Lunch   TIME: _____

FOOD: _____

_____

_____

DRINKS: _____

Dinner   TIME: _____

FOOD: _____

_____

_____

DRINKS: _____

Snacks/Other   TIME(S): _____

_____

_____

Supplements/Medications (if applicable)

_____

How many servings of vegetables did you eat today? —————————

Exercise

_____

Mindfulness practice

_____

List three things you are grateful for:

1. _____

2. _____

3. _____

What went well today?

_____

_____

_____

LET IT OUT

_____

_____

_____

_____

_____

DATE: / /

How are you feeling today?

UGH   OK   GOOD   AWESOME

How did you sleep last night?

Breakfast   TIME:

FOOD:

DRINKS:

Lunch   TIME:

FOOD:

DRINKS:

Dinner   TIME:

FOOD:

DRINKS:

Snacks/Other   TIME(S):

Supplements/Medications (if applicable)

_____

How many servings of vegetables did you eat today? _____

Exercise

_____

Mindfulness practice

_____

List three things you are grateful for:

1. _____

2. _____

3. _____

What went well today?

_____

_____

_____

LET IT OUT

_____

_____

_____

_____

_____

How are you feeling today?

UGH   OK   GOOD   AWESOME

How did you sleep last night?

_____

Breakfast   TIME: _____

FOOD: _____

_____

_____

DRINKS: _____

Lunch   TIME: _____

FOOD: _____

_____

_____

DRINKS: _____

Dinner   TIME: _____

FOOD: _____

_____

_____

DRINKS: _____

Snacks/Other   TIME(S): _____

_____

_____

Supplements/Medications (if applicable)

_____

How many servings of vegetables did you eat today? ——————————

Exercise

_____

Mindfulness practice

_____

List three things you are grateful for:

1. _____

2. _____

3. _____

What went well today?

_____

_____

_____

LET IT OUT

_____

_____

_____

_____

_____

DATE: /   /

How are you feeling today?

UGH   OK   GOOD   AWESOME

How did you sleep last night?

_____

Breakfast   TIME: _____

FOOD: _____

_____

_____

DRINKS: _____

Lunch   TIME: _____

FOOD: _____

_____

_____

DRINKS: _____

Dinner   TIME: _____

FOOD: _____

_____

_____

DRINKS: _____

Snacks/Other   TIME(S): _____

_____

_____

Supplements/Medications (if applicable)

_____

How many servings of vegetables did you eat today? _____

Exercise

_____

Mindfulness practice

_____

List three things you are grateful for:

1. _____

2. _____

3. _____

What went well today?

_____

_____

_____

LET IT OUT

_____

_____

_____

_____

_____

DATE: / /

How are you feeling today?

UGH   OK   GOOD   AWESOME

How did you sleep last night?

_____

Breakfast   TIME: _____

FOOD: _____

_____

_____

DRINKS: _____

Lunch   TIME: _____

FOOD: _____

_____

_____

DRINKS: _____

Dinner   TIME: _____

FOOD: _____

_____

_____

DRINKS: _____

Snacks/Other   TIME(S): _____

_____

_____

Supplements/Medications (if applicable)

_____

How many servings of vegetables did you eat today? _____

Exercise

_____

Mindfulness practice

_____

List three things you are grateful for:

1. _____

2. _____

3. _____

What went well today?

_____

_____

_____

LET IT OUT

_____

_____

_____

_____

_____

DATE: / /

How are you feeling today?

UGH   OK   GOOD   AWESOME

How did you sleep last night?

_____

Breakfast   TIME: _____

FOOD: _____

_____

_____

DRINKS: _____

Lunch   TIME: _____

FOOD: _____

_____

_____

DRINKS: _____

Dinner   TIME: _____

FOOD: _____

_____

_____

DRINKS: _____

Snacks/Other   TIME(S): _____

_____

_____

Supplements/Medications (if applicable)

_____

How many servings of vegetables did you eat today? _____

Exercise

_____

Mindfulness practice

_____

List three things you are grateful for:

1. _____

2. _____

3. _____

What went well today?

_____

_____

_____

LET IT OUT

_____

_____

_____

_____

_____

DATE: / /

How are you feeling today?

UGH   OK   GOOD   AWESOME

How did you sleep last night?

_____

Breakfast   TIME: _____

FOOD: _____

_____

_____

DRINKS: _____

Lunch   TIME: _____

FOOD: _____

_____

_____

DRINKS: _____

Dinner   TIME: _____

FOOD: _____

_____

_____

DRINKS: _____

Snacks/Other   TIME(S): _____

_____

_____

Supplements/Medications (if applicable)

_____

How many servings of vegetables did you eat today? _____

Exercise

_____

Mindfulness practice

_____

List three things you are grateful for:

1. _____

2. _____

3. _____

What went well today?

_____

_____

_____

LET IT OUT

_____

_____

_____

_____

_____

DATE: /   /

How are you feeling today?

UGH   OK   GOOD   AWESOME

How did you sleep last night?

_____

Breakfast   TIME: _____

FOOD: _____

_____

_____

DRINKS: _____

Lunch   TIME: _____

FOOD: _____

_____

_____

DRINKS: _____

Dinner   TIME: _____

FOOD: _____

_____

_____

DRINKS: _____

Snacks/Other   TIME(S): _____

_____

_____

Supplements/Medications (if applicable)

_____

How many servings of vegetables did you eat today? _____

Exercise

_____

Mindfulness practice

_____

List three things you are grateful for:

1. _____

2. _____

3. _____

What went well today?

_____

_____

_____

LET IT OUT

_____

_____

_____

_____

_____

DATE: /   /

How are you feeling today?

UGH   OK   GOOD   AWESOME

How did you sleep last night?

_____

Breakfast   TIME: _____

FOOD: _____

_____

_____

DRINKS: _____

Lunch   TIME: _____

FOOD: _____

_____

_____

DRINKS: _____

Dinner   TIME: _____

FOOD: _____

_____

_____

DRINKS: _____

Snacks/Other   TIME(S): _____

_____

_____

Supplements/Medications (if applicable)

_____

How many servings of vegetables did you eat today? ————————

Exercise

_____

Mindfulness practice

_____

List three things you are grateful for:

1. _____

2. _____

3. _____

What went well today?

_____

_____

_____

LET IT OUT

_____

_____

_____

_____

_____

DATE: /   /

How are you feeling today?

UGH   OK   GOOD   AWESOME

How did you sleep last night?

_____

Breakfast   TIME: _____

FOOD: _____

_____

_____

DRINKS: _____

Lunch   TIME: _____

FOOD: _____

_____

_____

DRINKS: _____

Dinner   TIME: _____

FOOD: _____

_____

_____

DRINKS: _____

Snacks/Other   TIME(S): _____

_____

_____

Supplements/Medications (if applicable)

_____

How many servings of vegetables did you eat today? ——————————

Exercise

_____

Mindfulness practice

_____

List three things you are grateful for:

1. _____

2. _____

3. _____

What went well today?

_____

_____

_____

LET IT OUT

_____

_____

_____

_____

_____

DATE: / /

How are you feeling today?

UGH   OK   GOOD   AWESOME

How did you sleep last night?

_____

Breakfast   TIME: _____

FOOD: _____

_____

_____

DRINKS: _____

Lunch   TIME: _____

FOOD: _____

_____

_____

DRINKS: _____

Dinner   TIME: _____

FOOD: _____

_____

_____

DRINKS: _____

Snacks/Other   TIME(S): _____

_____

_____

Supplements/Medications (if applicable)

_____

How many servings of vegetables did you eat today? _____

Exercise

_____

Mindfulness practice

_____

List three things you are grateful for:

1. _____

2. _____

3. _____

What went well today?

_____

_____

_____

LET IT OUT

_____

_____

_____

_____

_____

DATE: / /

How are you feeling today?

UGH　　　　OK　　　　GOOD　　　　AWESOME

How did you sleep last night?

Breakfast　　　TIME:

FOOD:

DRINKS:

Lunch　　　TIME:

FOOD:

DRINKS:

Dinner　　　TIME:

FOOD:

DRINKS:

Snacks/Other　　　TIME(S):

Supplements/Medications (if applicable)

_____

How many servings of vegetables did you eat today? _____

Exercise

_____

Mindfulness practice

_____

List three things you are grateful for:

1. _____

2. _____

3. _____

What went well today?

_____

_____

_____

LET IT OUT

_____

_____

_____

_____

_____

DATE: / /

How are you feeling today?

UGH   OK   GOOD   AWESOME

How did you sleep last night?

_____

Breakfast   TIME: _____

FOOD: _____

_____

_____

DRINKS: _____

Lunch   TIME: _____

FOOD: _____

_____

_____

DRINKS: _____

Dinner   TIME: _____

FOOD: _____

_____

_____

DRINKS: _____

Snacks/Other   TIME(S): _____

_____

_____

Supplements/Medications (if applicable)

_____

How many servings of vegetables did you eat today? _____

Exercise

_____

Mindfulness practice

_____

List three things you are grateful for:

1. _____

2. _____

3. _____

What went well today?

_____

_____

_____

LET IT OUT

_____

_____

_____

_____

_____

DATE: / /

How are you feeling today?

UGH   OK   GOOD   AWESOME

How did you sleep last night?

_____

Breakfast   TIME: _____

FOOD: _____

_____

_____

DRINKS: _____

Lunch   TIME: _____

FOOD: _____

_____

_____

DRINKS: _____

Dinner   TIME: _____

FOOD: _____

_____

_____

DRINKS: _____

Snacks/Other   TIME(S): _____

_____

_____

Supplements/Medications (if applicable)

_____

How many servings of vegetables did you eat today? ————————

Exercise

_____

Mindfulness practice

_____

List three things you are grateful for:

1._____

2._____

3._____

What went well today?

_____

_____

_____

LET IT OUT

_____

_____

_____

_____

_____

DATE: / /

How are you feeling today?

UGH   OK   GOOD   AWESOME

How did you sleep last night?

_____

Breakfast   TIME: _____

FOOD: _____

_____

_____

DRINKS: _____

Lunch   TIME: _____

FOOD: _____

_____

_____

DRINKS: _____

Dinner   TIME: _____

FOOD: _____

_____

_____

DRINKS: _____

Snacks/Other   TIME(S): _____

_____

_____

Supplements/Medications (if applicable)

_____

How many servings of vegetables did you eat today? _____

Exercise

_____

Mindfulness practice

_____

List three things you are grateful for:

1. _____

2. _____

3. _____

What went well today?

_____

_____

_____

LET IT OUT

_____

_____

_____

_____

_____

DATE: / /

How are you feeling today?

UGH   OK   GOOD   AWESOME

How did you sleep last night?

_____

Breakfast   TIME: _____

FOOD: _____

_____

_____

DRINKS: _____

Lunch   TIME: _____

FOOD: _____

_____

_____

DRINKS: _____

Dinner   TIME: _____

FOOD: _____

_____

_____

DRINKS: _____

Snacks/Other   TIME(S): _____

_____

_____

Supplements/Medications (if applicable)

_____

How many servings of vegetables did you eat today? ——————————

Exercise

_____

Mindfulness practice

_____

List three things you are grateful for:

1. _____

2. _____

3. _____

What went well today?

_____

_____

_____

LET IT OUT

_____

_____

_____

_____

_____

DATE: / /

How are you feeling today?

UGH   OK   GOOD   AWESOME

How did you sleep last night?

_____

Breakfast   TIME: _____

FOOD: _____

_____

_____

DRINKS: _____

Lunch   TIME: _____

FOOD: _____

_____

_____

DRINKS: _____

Dinner   TIME: _____

FOOD: _____

_____

_____

DRINKS: _____

Snacks/Other   TIME(S): _____

_____

_____

Supplements/Medications (if applicable)

_____

How many servings of vegetables did you eat today? _____

Exercise

_____

Mindfulness practice

_____

List three things you are grateful for:

1. _____

2. _____

3. _____

What went well today?

_____

_____

_____

LET IT OUT

_____

_____

_____

_____

_____

DATE: /   /

How are you feeling today?

UGH   OK   GOOD   AWESOME

How did you sleep last night?

_____

Breakfast   TIME: _____

FOOD: _____

_____

_____

DRINKS: _____

Lunch   TIME: _____

FOOD: _____

_____

_____

DRINKS: _____

Dinner   TIME: _____

FOOD: _____

_____

_____

DRINKS: _____

Snacks/Other   TIME(S): _____

_____

_____

Supplements/Medications (if applicable)

_____

How many servings of vegetables did you eat today? _____

Exercise

_____

Mindfulness practice

_____

List three things you are grateful for:

1. _____

2. _____

3. _____

What went well today?

_____

_____

_____

LET IT OUT

_____

_____

_____

_____

_____

DATE: / /

How are you feeling today?

UGH   OK   GOOD   AWESOME

How did you sleep last night?

_____

Breakfast   TIME: _____

FOOD: _____

_____

_____

DRINKS: _____

Lunch   TIME: _____

FOOD: _____

_____

_____

DRINKS: _____

Dinner   TIME: _____

FOOD: _____

_____

_____

DRINKS: _____

Snacks/Other   TIME(S): _____

_____

_____

Supplements/Medications (if applicable)

_____

How many servings of vegetables did you eat today? ———————————

Exercise

_____

Mindfulness practice

_____

List three things you are grateful for:

1. _____

2. _____

3. _____

What went well today?

_____

_____

_____

LET IT OUT

_____

_____

_____

_____

_____

DATE: / /

How are you feeling today?

UGH   OK   GOOD   AWESOME

How did you sleep last night?

_____

Breakfast   TIME: _____

FOOD: _____

_____

_____

DRINKS: _____

Lunch   TIME: _____

FOOD: _____

_____

_____

DRINKS: _____

Dinner   TIME: _____

FOOD: _____

_____

_____

DRINKS: _____

Snacks/Other   TIME(S): _____

_____

_____

Supplements/Medications (if applicable)

_____

How many servings of vegetables did you eat today? _____

Exercise

_____

Mindfulness practice

_____

List three things you are grateful for:

1. _____

2. _____

3. _____

What went well today?

_____

_____

_____

LET IT OUT

_____

_____

_____

_____

_____

DATE: / /

How are you feeling today?

UGH   OK   GOOD   AWESOME

How did you sleep last night?

_____

Breakfast   TIME: _____

FOOD: _____

_____

_____

DRINKS: _____

Lunch   TIME: _____

FOOD: _____

_____

_____

DRINKS: _____

Dinner   TIME: _____

FOOD: _____

_____

_____

DRINKS: _____

Snacks/Other   TIME(S): _____

_____

_____

Supplements/Medications (if applicable)

_____

How many servings of vegetables did you eat today? _____

Exercise

_____

Mindfulness practice

_____

List three things you are grateful for:

1. _____

2. _____

3. _____

What went well today?

_____

_____

_____

LET IT OUT

_____

_____

_____

_____

_____

DATE: / /

How are you feeling today?

UGH   OK   GOOD   AWESOME

How did you sleep last night?

_____

Breakfast   TIME: _____

FOOD: _____

_____

_____

DRINKS: _____

Lunch   TIME: _____

FOOD: _____

_____

_____

DRINKS: _____

Dinner   TIME: _____

FOOD: _____

_____

_____

DRINKS: _____

Snacks/Other   TIME(S): _____

_____

_____

Supplements/Medications (if applicable)

_____

How many servings of vegetables did you eat today? ——————————

Exercise

_____

Mindfulness practice

_____

List three things you are grateful for:

1. _____

2. _____

3. _____

What went well today?

_____

_____

_____

LET IT OUT

_____

_____

_____

_____

_____

DATE: /   /

How are you feeling today?

UGH   OK   GOOD   AWESOME

How did you sleep last night?

_____

Breakfast   TIME: _____

FOOD: _____

_____

_____

DRINKS: _____

Lunch   TIME: _____

FOOD: _____

_____

_____

DRINKS: _____

Dinner   TIME: _____

FOOD: _____

_____

_____

DRINKS: _____

Snacks/Other   TIME(S): _____

_____

_____

Supplements/Medications (if applicable)

_____

How many servings of vegetables did you eat today? _____

Exercise

_____

Mindfulness practice

_____

List three things you are grateful for:

1. _____

2. _____

3. _____

What went well today?

_____

_____

_____

LET IT OUT

_____

_____

_____

_____

DATE: / /

How are you feeling today?

UGH   OK   GOOD   AWESOME

How did you sleep last night?

_____

Breakfast   TIME: _____

FOOD: _____

_____

_____

DRINKS: _____

Lunch   TIME: _____

FOOD: _____

_____

_____

DRINKS: _____

Dinner   TIME: _____

FOOD: _____

_____

_____

DRINKS: _____

Snacks/Other   TIME(S): _____

_____

_____

Supplements/Medications (if applicable)

_____

How many servings of vegetables did you eat today? _____

Exercise

_____

Mindfulness practice

_____

List three things you are grateful for:

1. _____

2. _____

3. _____

What went well today?

_____

_____

_____

LET IT OUT

_____

_____

_____

_____

_____

DATE: / /

How are you feeling today?

UGH   OK   GOOD   AWESOME

How did you sleep last night?

_____

Breakfast   TIME: _____

FOOD: _____

_____

_____

DRINKS: _____

Lunch   TIME: _____

FOOD: _____

_____

_____

DRINKS: _____

Dinner   TIME: _____

FOOD: _____

_____

_____

DRINKS: _____

Snacks/Other   TIME(S): _____

_____

_____

Supplements/Medications (if applicable)

_____

How many servings of vegetables did you eat today? _____

Exercise

_____

Mindfulness practice

_____

List three things you are grateful for:

1. _____

2. _____

3. _____

What went well today?

_____

_____

_____

LET IT OUT

_____

_____

_____

_____

_____

DATE: / /

How are you feeling today?

UGH   OK   GOOD   AWESOME

How did you sleep last night?

_____

Breakfast   TIME: _____

FOOD: _____

_____

_____

DRINKS: _____

Lunch   TIME: _____

FOOD: _____

_____

_____

DRINKS: _____

Dinner   TIME: _____

FOOD: _____

_____

_____

DRINKS: _____

Snacks/Other   TIME(S): _____

_____

_____

Supplements/Medications (if applicable)

_____

How many servings of vegetables did you eat today? ——————————

Exercise

_____

Mindfulness practice

_____

List three things you are grateful for:

1. _____

2. _____

3. _____

What went well today?

_____

_____

_____

LET IT OUT

_____

_____

_____

_____

_____

DATE: / /

How are you feeling today?

UGH   OK   GOOD   AWESOME

How did you sleep last night?

_____

Breakfast   TIME: _____

FOOD: _____

_____

_____

DRINKS: _____

Lunch   TIME: _____

FOOD: _____

_____

_____

DRINKS: _____

Dinner   TIME: _____

FOOD: _____

_____

_____

DRINKS: _____

Snacks/Other   TIME(S): _____

_____

_____

Supplements/Medications (if applicable)

_____

How many servings of vegetables did you eat today? _____

Exercise

_____

Mindfulness practice

_____

List three things you are grateful for:

1. _____

2. _____

3. _____

What went well today?

_____

_____

_____

LET IT OUT

_____

_____

_____

_____

_____

DATE: /   /

How are you feeling today?

UGH   OK   GOOD   AWESOME

How did you sleep last night?

_____

Breakfast   TIME: _____

FOOD: _____

_____

_____

DRINKS: _____

Lunch   TIME: _____

FOOD: _____

_____

_____

DRINKS: _____

Dinner   TIME: _____

FOOD: _____

_____

_____

DRINKS: _____

Snacks/Other   TIME(S): _____

_____

_____

Supplements/Medications (if applicable)

_____

How many servings of vegetables did you eat today? _____

Exercise

_____

Mindfulness practice

_____

List three things you are grateful for:

1. _____

2. _____

3. _____

What went well today?

_____

_____

_____

LET IT OUT

_____

_____

_____

_____

_____

DATE: /   /

How are you feeling today?

UGH   OK   GOOD   AWESOME

How did you sleep last night?

_____

Breakfast   TIME: _____

FOOD: _____

_____

_____

DRINKS: _____

Lunch   TIME: _____

FOOD: _____

_____

_____

DRINKS: _____

Dinner   TIME: _____

FOOD: _____

_____

_____

DRINKS: _____

Snacks/Other   TIME(S): _____

_____

_____

Supplements/Medications (if applicable)

_____

How many servings of vegetables did you eat today? _____

Exercise

_____

Mindfulness practice

_____

List three things you are grateful for:

1. _____

2. _____

3. _____

What went well today?

_____

_____

_____

LET IT OUT

_____

_____

_____

_____

_____

DATE: / /

How are you feeling today?

UGH   OK   GOOD   AWESOME

How did you sleep last night?

_____

Breakfast   TIME: _____

FOOD: _____

_____

_____

DRINKS: _____

Lunch   TIME: _____

FOOD: _____

_____

_____

DRINKS: _____

Dinner   TIME: _____

FOOD: _____

_____

_____

DRINKS: _____

Snacks/Other   TIME(S): _____

_____

_____

Supplements/Medications (if applicable)

_____

How many servings of vegetables did you eat today? ————————————

Exercise

_____

Mindfulness practice

_____

List three things you are grateful for:

1. _____

2. _____

3. _____

What went well today?

_____

_____

_____

LET IT OUT

_____

_____

_____

_____

_____

DATE: / /

How are you feeling today?

UGH   OK   GOOD   AWESOME

How did you sleep last night?

_____

Breakfast   TIME: _____

FOOD: _____

_____

_____

DRINKS: _____

Lunch   TIME: _____

FOOD: _____

_____

_____

DRINKS: _____

Dinner   TIME: _____

FOOD: _____

_____

_____

DRINKS: _____

Snacks/Other   TIME(S): _____

_____

_____

Supplements/Medications (if applicable)

_____

How many servings of vegetables did you eat today? _____

Exercise

_____

Mindfulness practice

_____

List three things you are grateful for:

1. _____

2. _____

3. _____

What went well today?

_____

_____

_____

LET IT OUT

_____

_____

_____

_____

_____

DATE: / /

How are you feeling today?

UGH   OK   GOOD   AWESOME

How did you sleep last night?

_____

Breakfast   TIME: _____

FOOD: _____

_____

_____

DRINKS: _____

Lunch   TIME: _____

FOOD: _____

_____

_____

DRINKS: _____

Dinner   TIME: _____

FOOD: _____

_____

_____

DRINKS: _____

Snacks/Other   TIME(S): _____

_____

_____

Supplements/Medications (if applicable)

_____

How many servings of vegetables did you eat today? _____

Exercise

_____

Mindfulness practice

_____

List three things you are grateful for:

1. _____

2. _____

3. _____

What went well today?

_____

_____

_____

LET IT OUT

_____

_____

_____

_____

_____

DATE: / /

How are you feeling today?

UGH   OK   GOOD   AWESOME

How did you sleep last night?

_____

Breakfast   TIME: _____

FOOD: _____

_____

_____

DRINKS: _____

Lunch   TIME: _____

FOOD: _____

_____

_____

DRINKS: _____

Dinner   TIME: _____

FOOD: _____

_____

_____

DRINKS: _____

Snacks/Other   TIME(S): _____

_____

_____

Supplements/Medications (if applicable)

_____

How many servings of vegetables did you eat today? _____

Exercise

_____

Mindfulness practice

_____

List three things you are grateful for:

1. _____

2. _____

3. _____

What went well today?

_____

_____

_____

LET IT OUT

_____

_____

_____

_____

_____

DATE: / /

How are you feeling today?

UGH   OK   GOOD   AWESOME

How did you sleep last night?

_____

Breakfast   TIME: _____

FOOD: _____

_____

_____

DRINKS: _____

Lunch   TIME: _____

FOOD: _____

_____

_____

DRINKS: _____

Dinner   TIME: _____

FOOD: _____

_____

_____

DRINKS: _____

Snacks/Other   TIME(S): _____

_____

_____

Supplements/Medications (if applicable)

_____

How many servings of vegetables did you eat today? _____

Exercise

_____

Mindfulness practice

_____

List three things you are grateful for:

1. _____

2. _____

3. _____

What went well today?

_____

_____

_____

LET IT OUT

_____

_____

_____

_____

_____

DATE: /   /

How are you feeling today?

UGH   OK   GOOD   AWESOME

How did you sleep last night?

_____

Breakfast   TIME: _____

FOOD: _____

_____

_____

DRINKS: _____

Lunch   TIME: _____

FOOD: _____

_____

_____

DRINKS: _____

Dinner   TIME: _____

FOOD: _____

_____

_____

DRINKS: _____

Snacks/Other   TIME(S): _____

_____

_____

Supplements/Medications (if applicable)

_____

How many servings of vegetables did you eat today? ——————————

Exercise

_____

Mindfulness practice

_____

List three things you are grateful for:

1. _____

2. _____

3. _____

What went well today?

_____

_____

_____

LET IT OUT

_____

_____

_____

_____

_____

DATE: /   /

How are you feeling today?

UGH   OK   GOOD   AWESOME

How did you sleep last night?

_____

Breakfast   TIME: _____

FOOD: _____

_____

_____

DRINKS: _____

Lunch   TIME: _____

FOOD: _____

_____

_____

DRINKS: _____

Dinner   TIME: _____

FOOD: _____

_____

_____

DRINKS: _____

Snacks/Other   TIME(S): _____

_____

_____

Supplements/Medications (if applicable)

_____

How many servings of vegetables did you eat today? ———————————

Exercise

_____

Mindfulness practice

_____

List three things you are grateful for:

1. _____

2. _____

3. _____

What went well today?

_____

_____

_____

LET IT OUT

_____

_____

_____

_____

_____

DATE: /   /

How are you feeling today?

UGH   OK   GOOD   AWESOME

How did you sleep last night?

_____

Breakfast   TIME: _____

FOOD: _____

_____

_____

DRINKS: _____

Lunch   TIME: _____

FOOD: _____

_____

_____

DRINKS: _____

Dinner   TIME: _____

FOOD: _____

_____

_____

DRINKS: _____

Snacks/Other   TIME(S): _____

_____

_____

Supplements/Medications (if applicable)

_____

How many servings of vegetables did you eat today? ———————————

Exercise

_____

Mindfulness practice

_____

List three things you are grateful for:

1. _____

2. _____

3. _____

What went well today?

_____

_____

_____

LET IT OUT

_____

_____

_____

_____

_____

DATE: /   /

How are you feeling today?

UGH   OK   GOOD   AWESOME

How did you sleep last night?

_____

Breakfast   TIME: _____

FOOD: _____

_____

_____

DRINKS: _____

Lunch   TIME: _____

FOOD: _____

_____

_____

DRINKS: _____

Dinner   TIME: _____

FOOD: _____

_____

_____

DRINKS: _____

Snacks/Other   TIME(S): _____

_____

_____

Supplements/Medications (if applicable)

_____

How many servings of vegetables did you eat today? ——————————

Exercise

_____

Mindfulness practice

_____

List three things you are grateful for:

1. _____

2. _____

3. _____

What went well today?

_____

_____

_____

LET IT OUT

_____

_____

_____

_____

_____

DATE: / /

How are you feeling today?

UGH   OK   GOOD   AWESOME

How did you sleep last night?

_____

Breakfast   TIME: _____

FOOD: _____

_____

_____

DRINKS: _____

Lunch   TIME: _____

FOOD: _____

_____

_____

DRINKS: _____

Dinner   TIME: _____

FOOD: _____

_____

_____

DRINKS: _____

Snacks/Other   TIME(S): _____

_____

_____

Supplements/Medications (if applicable)

_____

How many servings of vegetables did you eat today? _____

Exercise

_____

Mindfulness practice

_____

List three things you are grateful for:

1. _____

2. _____

3. _____

What went well today?

_____

_____

_____

LET IT OUT

_____

_____

_____

_____

DATE: / /

How are you feeling today?

UGH   OK   GOOD   AWESOME

How did you sleep last night?

_____

Breakfast   TIME: _____

FOOD: _____

_____

_____

DRINKS: _____

Lunch   TIME: _____

FOOD: _____

_____

_____

DRINKS: _____

Dinner   TIME: _____

FOOD: _____

_____

_____

DRINKS: _____

Snacks/Other   TIME(S): _____

_____

_____

Supplements/Medications (if applicable)

_____

How many servings of vegetables did you eat today? ——————————

Exercise

_____

Mindfulness practice

_____

List three things you are grateful for:

1. _____

2. _____

3. _____

What went well today?

_____

_____

_____

LET IT OUT

_____

_____

_____

_____

_____

DATE: / /

How are you feeling today?

UGH   OK   GOOD   AWESOME

How did you sleep last night?

_____

Breakfast   TIME: _____

FOOD: _____

_____

_____

DRINKS: _____

Lunch   TIME: _____

FOOD: _____

_____

_____

DRINKS: _____

Dinner   TIME: _____

FOOD: _____

_____

_____

DRINKS: _____

Snacks/Other   TIME(S): _____

_____

_____

Supplements/Medications (if applicable)

_____

How many servings of vegetables did you eat today? _____

Exercise

_____

Mindfulness practice

_____

List three things you are grateful for:

1. _____

2. _____

3. _____

What went well today?

_____

_____

_____

LET IT OUT

_____

_____

_____

_____

_____

DATE: / /

How are you feeling today?

UGH   OK   GOOD   AWESOME

How did you sleep last night?

_____

Breakfast   TIME: _____

FOOD: _____

_____

_____

DRINKS: _____

Lunch   TIME: _____

FOOD: _____

_____

_____

DRINKS: _____

Dinner   TIME: _____

FOOD: _____

_____

_____

DRINKS: _____

Snacks/Other   TIME(S): _____

_____

_____

Supplements/Medications (if applicable)

_____

How many servings of vegetables did you eat today? _____

Exercise

_____

Mindfulness practice

_____

List three things you are grateful for:

1. _____

2. _____

3. _____

What went well today?

_____

_____

_____

LET IT OUT

_____

_____

_____

_____

_____

DATE: / /

How are you feeling today?

UGH   OK   GOOD   AWESOME

How did you sleep last night?

_____

Breakfast   TIME: _____

FOOD: _____

_____

_____

DRINKS: _____

Lunch   TIME: _____

FOOD: _____

_____

_____

DRINKS: _____

Dinner   TIME: _____

FOOD: _____

_____

_____

DRINKS: _____

Snacks/Other   TIME(S): _____

_____

_____

Supplements/Medications (if applicable)

_____

How many servings of vegetables did you eat today? _____

Exercise

_____

Mindfulness practice

_____

List three things you are grateful for:

1. _____

2. _____

3. _____

What went well today?

_____

_____

_____

LET IT OUT

_____

_____

_____

_____

_____

DATE: / /

How are you feeling today?

UGH   OK   GOOD   AWESOME

How did you sleep last night?

_____

Breakfast   TIME: _____

FOOD: _____

_____

_____

DRINKS: _____

Lunch   TIME: _____

FOOD: _____

_____

_____

DRINKS: _____

Dinner   TIME: _____

FOOD: _____

_____

_____

DRINKS: _____

Snacks/Other   TIME(S): _____

_____

_____

Supplements/Medications (if applicable)

_____

How many servings of vegetables did you eat today? ——————————

Exercise

_____

Mindfulness practice

_____

List three things you are grateful for:

1. _____

2. _____

3. _____

What went well today?

_____

_____

_____

LET IT OUT

_____

_____

_____

_____

_____

DATE: /   /

How are you feeling today?

UGH   OK   GOOD   AWESOME

How did you sleep last night?

_____

Breakfast   TIME: _____

FOOD: _____

_____

_____

DRINKS: _____

Lunch   TIME: _____

FOOD: _____

_____

_____

DRINKS: _____

Dinner   TIME: _____

FOOD: _____

_____

_____

DRINKS: _____

Snacks/Other   TIME(S): _____

_____

_____

Supplements/Medications (if applicable)

_____

How many servings of vegetables did you eat today? _____

Exercise

_____

Mindfulness practice

_____

List three things you are grateful for:

1. _____

2. _____

3. _____

What went well today?

_____

_____

_____

LET IT OUT

_____

_____

_____

_____

_____

DATE: / /

How are you feeling today?

UGH   OK   GOOD   AWESOME

How did you sleep last night?

_____

Breakfast   TIME: _____

FOOD: _____

_____

_____

DRINKS: _____

Lunch   TIME: _____

FOOD: _____

_____

_____

DRINKS: _____

Dinner   TIME: _____

FOOD: _____

_____

_____

DRINKS: _____

Snacks/Other   TIME(S): _____

_____

_____

Supplements/Medications (if applicable)

_____

How many servings of vegetables did you eat today? ——————————

Exercise

_____

Mindfulness practice

_____

List three things you are grateful for:

1. _____

2. _____

3. _____

What went well today?

_____

_____

_____

LET IT OUT

_____

_____

_____

_____

_____

DATE: / /

How are you feeling today?

UGH   OK   GOOD   AWESOME

How did you sleep last night?

_____

Breakfast   TIME: _____

FOOD: _____

_____

_____

DRINKS: _____

Lunch   TIME: _____

FOOD: _____

_____

_____

DRINKS: _____

Dinner   TIME: _____

FOOD: _____

_____

_____

DRINKS: _____

Snacks/Other   TIME(S): _____

_____

_____

Supplements/Medications (if applicable)

_____

How many servings of vegetables did you eat today? ———————————

Exercise

_____

Mindfulness practice

_____

List three things you are grateful for:

1. _____

2. _____

3. _____

What went well today?

_____

_____

_____

LET IT OUT

_____

_____

_____

_____

DATE: / /

How are you feeling today?

UGH   OK   GOOD   AWESOME

How did you sleep last night?

_____

Breakfast   TIME: _____

FOOD: _____

_____

_____

DRINKS: _____

Lunch   TIME: _____

FOOD: _____

_____

_____

DRINKS: _____

Dinner   TIME: _____

FOOD: _____

_____

_____

DRINKS: _____

Snacks/Other   TIME(S): _____

_____

_____

Supplements/Medications (if applicable)

_____

How many servings of vegetables did you eat today? _____

Exercise

_____

Mindfulness practice

_____

List three things you are grateful for:

1. _____

2. _____

3. _____

What went well today?

_____

_____

_____

LET IT OUT

_____

_____

_____

_____

_____

DATE: /   /

How are you feeling today?

UGH   OK   GOOD   AWESOME

How did you sleep last night?

_____

Breakfast   TIME: _____

FOOD: _____

_____

_____

DRINKS: _____

Lunch   TIME: _____

FOOD: _____

_____

_____

DRINKS: _____

Dinner   TIME: _____

FOOD: _____

_____

_____

DRINKS: _____

Snacks/Other   TIME(S): _____

_____

_____

Supplements/Medications (if applicable)

_____

How many servings of vegetables did you eat today? ————————

Exercise

_____

Mindfulness practice

_____

List three things you are grateful for:

1. _____

2. _____

3. _____

What went well today?

_____

_____

_____

LET IT OUT

_____

_____

_____

_____

_____

DATE: /   /

How are you feeling today?

UGH   OK   GOOD   AWESOME

How did you sleep last night?

_____

Breakfast   TIME: _____

FOOD: _____

_____

_____

DRINKS: _____

Lunch   TIME: _____

FOOD: _____

_____

_____

DRINKS: _____

Dinner   TIME: _____

FOOD: _____

_____

_____

DRINKS: _____

Snacks/Other   TIME(S): _____

_____

_____

Supplements/Medications (if applicable)

_____

How many servings of vegetables did you eat today? _____

Exercise

_____

Mindfulness practice

_____

List three things you are grateful for:

1. _____

2. _____

3. _____

What went well today?

_____

_____

_____

LET IT OUT

_____

_____

_____

_____

_____

DATE: / /

How are you feeling today?

UGH   OK   GOOD   AWESOME

How did you sleep last night?

_____

Breakfast   TIME: _____

FOOD: _____

_____

_____

DRINKS: _____

Lunch   TIME: _____

FOOD: _____

_____

_____

DRINKS: _____

Dinner   TIME: _____

FOOD: _____

_____

_____

DRINKS: _____

Snacks/Other   TIME(S): _____

_____

_____

Supplements/Medications (if applicable)

_____

How many servings of vegetables did you eat today? _____

Exercise

_____

Mindfulness practice

_____

List three things you are grateful for:

1. _____

2. _____

3. _____

What went well today?

_____

_____

_____

LET IT OUT

_____

_____

_____

_____

_____

DATE: / /

How are you feeling today?

UGH   OK   GOOD   AWESOME

How did you sleep last night?

_____

Breakfast   TIME: _____

FOOD: _____

_____

_____

DRINKS: _____

Lunch   TIME: _____

FOOD: _____

_____

_____

DRINKS: _____

Dinner   TIME: _____

FOOD: _____

_____

_____

DRINKS: _____

Snacks/Other   TIME(S): _____

_____

_____

Supplements/Medications (if applicable)

_____

How many servings of vegetables did you eat today? _____

Exercise

_____

Mindfulness practice

_____

List three things you are grateful for:

1. _____

2. _____

3. _____

What went well today?

_____

_____

_____

LET IT OUT

_____

_____

_____

_____

_____

DATE: / /

How are you feeling today?

UGH   OK   GOOD   AWESOME

How did you sleep last night?

_____

Breakfast   TIME: _____

FOOD: _____

_____

_____

DRINKS: _____

Lunch   TIME: _____

FOOD: _____

_____

_____

DRINKS: _____

Dinner   TIME: _____

FOOD: _____

_____

_____

DRINKS: _____

Snacks/Other   TIME(S): _____

_____

_____

Supplements/Medications (if applicable)

_____

How many servings of vegetables did you eat today? _____

Exercise

_____

Mindfulness practice

_____

List three things you are grateful for:

1. _____

2. _____

3. _____

What went well today?

_____

_____

_____

LET IT OUT

_____

_____

_____

_____

_____

DATE: / /

How are you feeling today?

UGH   OK   GOOD   AWESOME

How did you sleep last night?

_____

Breakfast   TIME:

FOOD:

_____

_____

DRINKS:

Lunch   TIME:

FOOD:

_____

_____

DRINKS:

Dinner   TIME:

FOOD:

_____

_____

DRINKS:

Snacks/Other   TIME(S):

_____

_____

Supplements/Medications (if applicable)

_____

How many servings of vegetables did you eat today? ————————

Exercise

_____

Mindfulness practice

_____

List three things you are grateful for:

1. _____

2. _____

3. _____

What went well today?

_____

_____

_____

LET IT OUT

_____

_____

_____

_____

_____

DATE: / /

How are you feeling today?

UGH   OK   GOOD   AWESOME

How did you sleep last night?

_____

Breakfast   TIME: _____

FOOD: _____

_____

_____

DRINKS: _____

Lunch   TIME: _____

FOOD: _____

_____

_____

DRINKS: _____

Dinner   TIME: _____

FOOD: _____

_____

_____

DRINKS: _____

Snacks/Other   TIME(S): _____

_____

_____

Supplements/Medications (if applicable)

_____

How many servings of vegetables did you eat today? _____

Exercise

_____

Mindfulness practice

_____

List three things you are grateful for:

1. _____

2. _____

3. _____

What went well today?

_____

_____

_____

LET IT OUT

_____

_____

_____

_____

_____

DATE: /   /

How are you feeling today?

UGH   OK   GOOD   AWESOME

How did you sleep last night?

_____

Breakfast   TIME: _____

FOOD: _____

_____

_____

DRINKS: _____

Lunch   TIME: _____

FOOD: _____

_____

_____

DRINKS: _____

Dinner   TIME: _____

FOOD: _____

_____

_____

DRINKS: _____

Snacks/Other   TIME(S): _____

_____

_____

Supplements/Medications (if applicable)

_____

How many servings of vegetables did you eat today? _____

Exercise

_____

Mindfulness practice

_____

List three things you are grateful for:

1. _____

2. _____

3. _____

What went well today?

_____

_____

_____

LET IT OUT

_____

_____

_____

_____

_____

DATE: /   /

How are you feeling today?

UGH   OK   GOOD   AWESOME

How did you sleep last night?

_____

Breakfast   TIME: _____

FOOD: _____

_____

_____

DRINKS: _____

Lunch   TIME: _____

FOOD: _____

_____

_____

DRINKS: _____

Dinner   TIME: _____

FOOD: _____

_____

_____

DRINKS: _____

Snacks/Other   TIME(S): _____

_____

_____

Supplements/Medications (if applicable)

_____

How many servings of vegetables did you eat today? _____

Exercise

_____

Mindfulness practice

_____

List three things you are grateful for:

1. _____

2. _____

3. _____

What went well today?

_____

_____

_____

LET IT OUT

_____

_____

_____

_____

_____

DATE: / /

How are you feeling today?

UGH   OK   GOOD   AWESOME

How did you sleep last night?

_____

Breakfast   TIME: _____

FOOD: _____

_____

_____

DRINKS: _____

Lunch   TIME: _____

FOOD: _____

_____

_____

DRINKS: _____

Dinner   TIME: _____

FOOD: _____

_____

_____

DRINKS: _____

Snacks/Other   TIME(S): _____

_____

_____

Supplements/Medications (if applicable)

_____

How many servings of vegetables did you eat today? _____

Exercise

_____

Mindfulness practice

_____

List three things you are grateful for:

1. _____

2. _____

3. _____

What went well today?

_____

_____

_____

LET IT OUT

_____

_____

_____

_____

_____

DATE: /   /

How are you feeling today?

UGH   OK   GOOD   AWESOME

How did you sleep last night?

_____

Breakfast   TIME: _____

FOOD: _____

_____

_____

DRINKS: _____

Lunch   TIME: _____

FOOD: _____

_____

_____

DRINKS: _____

Dinner   TIME: _____

FOOD: _____

_____

_____

DRINKS: _____

Snacks/Other   TIME(S): _____

_____

_____

Supplements/Medications (if applicable)

_____

How many servings of vegetables did you eat today? ——————————

Exercise

_____

Mindfulness practice

_____

List three things you are grateful for:

1. _____

2. _____

3. _____

What went well today?

_____

_____

_____

LET IT OUT

_____

_____

_____

_____

_____

DATE: / /

How are you feeling today?

UGH   OK   GOOD   AWESOME

How did you sleep last night?

_____

Breakfast   TIME: _____

FOOD: _____

_____

_____

DRINKS: _____

Lunch   TIME: _____

FOOD: _____

_____

_____

DRINKS: _____

Dinner   TIME: _____

FOOD: _____

_____

_____

DRINKS: _____

Snacks/Other   TIME(S): _____

_____

_____

Supplements/Medications (if applicable)

_____

How many servings of vegetables did you eat today? —————————

Exercise

_____

Mindfulness practice

_____

List three things you are grateful for:

1. _____

2. _____

3. _____

What went well today?

_____

_____

_____

LET IT OUT

_____

_____

_____

_____

_____

DATE: / /

How are you feeling today?

UGH   OK   GOOD   AWESOME

How did you sleep last night?

_____

Breakfast   TIME: _____

FOOD: _____

_____

_____

DRINKS: _____

Lunch   TIME: _____

FOOD: _____

_____

_____

DRINKS: _____

Dinner   TIME: _____

FOOD: _____

_____

_____

DRINKS: _____

Snacks/Other   TIME(S): _____

_____

_____

Supplements/Medications (if applicable)

_____

How many servings of vegetables did you eat today? _____

Exercise

_____

Mindfulness practice

_____

List three things you are grateful for:

1. _____

2. _____

3. _____

What went well today?

_____

_____

_____

LET IT OUT

_____

_____

_____

_____

_____

DATE: /   /

How are you feeling today?

UGH   OK   GOOD   AWESOME

How did you sleep last night?

_____

Breakfast   TIME: _____

FOOD: _____

_____

_____

DRINKS: _____

Lunch   TIME: _____

FOOD: _____

_____

_____

DRINKS: _____

Dinner   TIME: _____

FOOD: _____

_____

_____

DRINKS: _____

Snacks/Other   TIME(S): _____

_____

_____

Supplements/Medications (if applicable)

_____

How many servings of vegetables did you eat today? _____

Exercise

_____

Mindfulness practice

_____

List three things you are grateful for:

1. _____

2. _____

3. _____

What went well today?

_____

_____

_____

LET IT OUT

_____

_____

_____

_____

_____

DATE: /   /

How are you feeling today?

UGH   OK   GOOD   AWESOME

How did you sleep last night?

_____

Breakfast   TIME: _____

FOOD: _____

_____

_____

DRINKS: _____

Lunch   TIME: _____

FOOD: _____

_____

_____

DRINKS: _____

Dinner   TIME: _____

FOOD: _____

_____

_____

DRINKS: _____

Snacks/Other   TIME(S): _____

_____

_____

Supplements/Medications (if applicable)

_____

How many servings of vegetables did you eat today? ————————————

Exercise

_____

Mindfulness practice

_____

List three things you are grateful for:

1. _____

2. _____

3. _____

What went well today?

_____

_____

_____

LET IT OUT

_____

_____

_____

_____

DATE: / /

How are you feeling today?

UGH   OK   GOOD   AWESOME

How did you sleep last night?

_____

Breakfast   TIME: _____

FOOD: _____

_____

_____

DRINKS: _____

Lunch   TIME: _____

FOOD: _____

_____

_____

DRINKS: _____

Dinner   TIME: _____

FOOD: _____

_____

_____

DRINKS: _____

Snacks/Other   TIME(S): _____

_____

_____

Supplements/Medications (if applicable)

_____

How many servings of vegetables did you eat today? ————————————

Exercise

_____

Mindfulness practice

_____

List three things you are grateful for:

1. _____

2. _____

3. _____

What went well today?

_____

_____

_____

LET IT OUT

_____

_____

_____

_____

_____

DATE: / /

How are you feeling today?

UGH   OK   GOOD   AWESOME

How did you sleep last night?

_____

Breakfast   TIME: _____

FOOD: _____

_____

_____

DRINKS: _____

Lunch   TIME: _____

FOOD: _____

_____

_____

DRINKS: _____

Dinner   TIME: _____

FOOD: _____

_____

_____

DRINKS: _____

Snacks/Other   TIME(S): _____

_____

_____

Supplements/Medications (if applicable)

_____

How many servings of vegetables did you eat today? _____

Exercise

_____

Mindfulness practice

_____

List three things you are grateful for:

1. _____

2. _____

3. _____

What went well today?

_____

_____

_____

LET IT OUT

_____

_____

_____

_____

_____

DATE: / /

How are you feeling today?

UGH   OK   GOOD   AWESOME

How did you sleep last night?

_____

Breakfast   TIME: _____

FOOD: _____

_____

_____

DRINKS: _____

Lunch   TIME: _____

FOOD: _____

_____

_____

DRINKS: _____

Dinner   TIME: _____

FOOD: _____

_____

_____

DRINKS: _____

Snacks/Other   TIME(S): _____

_____

_____

Supplements/Medications (if applicable)

_____

How many servings of vegetables did you eat today? ————————

Exercise

_____

Mindfulness practice

_____

List three things you are grateful for:

1. _____

2. _____

3. _____

What went well today?

_____

_____

_____

LET IT OUT

_____

_____

_____

_____

_____

DATE: /   /

How are you feeling today?

UGH   OK   GOOD   AWESOME

How did you sleep last night?

_____

Breakfast   TIME: _____

FOOD: _____

_____

_____

DRINKS: _____

Lunch   TIME: _____

FOOD: _____

_____

_____

DRINKS: _____

Dinner   TIME: _____

FOOD: _____

_____

_____

DRINKS: _____

Snacks/Other   TIME(S): _____

_____

_____

Supplements/Medications (if applicable)

_____

How many servings of vegetables did you eat today? _____

Exercise

_____

Mindfulness practice

_____

List three things you are grateful for:

1. _____

2. _____

3. _____

What went well today?

_____

_____

_____

LET IT OUT

_____

_____

_____

_____

_____

DATE: /   /

How are you feeling today?

UGH   OK   GOOD   AWESOME

How did you sleep last night?

_____

Breakfast   TIME: _____

FOOD: _____

_____

_____

DRINKS: _____

Lunch   TIME: _____

FOOD: _____

_____

_____

DRINKS: _____

Dinner   TIME: _____

FOOD: _____

_____

_____

DRINKS: _____

Snacks/Other   TIME(S): _____

_____

_____

Supplements/Medications (if applicable)

_____

How many servings of vegetables did you eat today? _____

Exercise

_____

Mindfulness practice

_____

List three things you are grateful for:

1. _____

2. _____

3. _____

What went well today?

_____

_____

_____

LET IT OUT

_____

_____

_____

_____

_____

DATE: / /

How are you feeling today?

UGH   OK   GOOD   AWESOME

How did you sleep last night?

_____

Breakfast   TIME: _____

FOOD: _____

_____

_____

DRINKS: _____

Lunch   TIME: _____

FOOD: _____

_____

_____

DRINKS: _____

Dinner   TIME: _____

FOOD: _____

_____

_____

DRINKS: _____

Snacks/Other   TIME(S): _____

_____

_____

Supplements/Medications (if applicable)

_____

How many servings of vegetables did you eat today? ―――――――――――

Exercise

_____

Mindfulness practice

_____

List three things you are grateful for:

1. _____

2. _____

3. _____

What went well today?

_____

_____

_____

LET IT OUT

_____

_____

_____

_____

_____

DATE: / /

How are you feeling today?

UGH   OK   GOOD   AWESOME

How did you sleep last night?

_____

Breakfast   TIME: _____

FOOD: _____

_____

_____

DRINKS: _____

Lunch   TIME: _____

FOOD: _____

_____

_____

DRINKS: _____

Dinner   TIME: _____

FOOD: _____

_____

_____

DRINKS: _____

Snacks/Other   TIME(S): _____

_____

_____

Supplements/Medications (if applicable)

_____

How many servings of vegetables did you eat today? _____

Exercise

_____

Mindfulness practice

_____

List three things you are grateful for:

1. _____

2. _____

3. _____

What went well today?

_____

_____

_____

LET IT OUT

_____

_____

_____

_____

_____

DATE: /   /

How are you feeling today?

UGH   OK   GOOD   AWESOME

How did you sleep last night?

_____

Breakfast   TIME: _____

FOOD: _____

_____

_____

DRINKS: _____

Lunch   TIME: _____

FOOD: _____

_____

_____

DRINKS: _____

Dinner   TIME: _____

FOOD: _____

_____

_____

DRINKS: _____

Snacks/Other   TIME(S): _____

_____

_____

Supplements/Medications (if applicable)

_____

How many servings of vegetables did you eat today? _____

Exercise

_____

Mindfulness practice

_____

List three things you are grateful for:

1. _____

2. _____

3. _____

What went well today?

_____

_____

_____

LET IT OUT

_____

_____

_____

_____

_____

DATE: / /

How are you feeling today?

UGH   OK   GOOD   AWESOME

How did you sleep last night?

_____

Breakfast   TIME: _____

FOOD: _____

_____

_____

DRINKS: _____

Lunch   TIME: _____

FOOD: _____

_____

_____

DRINKS: _____

Dinner   TIME: _____

FOOD: _____

_____

_____

DRINKS: _____

Snacks/Other   TIME(S): _____

_____

_____

Supplements/Medications (if applicable)

_____

How many servings of vegetables did you eat today? _____

Exercise

_____

Mindfulness practice

_____

List three things you are grateful for:

1. _____

2. _____

3. _____

What went well today?

_____

_____

_____

LET IT OUT

_____

_____

_____

_____

_____

DATE: / /

How are you feeling today?

UGH   OK   GOOD   AWESOME

How did you sleep last night?

_____

Breakfast   TIME: _____

FOOD: _____

_____

_____

DRINKS: _____

Lunch   TIME: _____

FOOD: _____

_____

_____

DRINKS: _____

Dinner   TIME: _____

FOOD: _____

_____

_____

DRINKS: _____

Snacks/Other   TIME(S): _____

_____

_____

Supplements/Medications (if applicable)

_____

How many servings of vegetables did you eat today? _____

Exercise

_____

Mindfulness practice

_____

List three things you are grateful for:

1. _____

2. _____

3. _____

What went well today?

_____

_____

_____

LET IT OUT

_____

_____

_____

_____

_____

DATE: / /

How are you feeling today?

UGH   OK   GOOD   AWESOME

How did you sleep last night?

_____

Breakfast   TIME: _____

FOOD: _____

_____

_____

DRINKS: _____

Lunch   TIME: _____

FOOD: _____

_____

_____

DRINKS: _____

Dinner   TIME: _____

FOOD: _____

_____

_____

DRINKS: _____

Snacks/Other   TIME(S): _____

_____

_____

Supplements/Medications (if applicable)

_____

How many servings of vegetables did you eat today? _____

Exercise

_____

Mindfulness practice

_____

List three things you are grateful for:

1. _____

2. _____

3. _____

What went well today?

_____

_____

_____

LET IT OUT

_____

_____

_____

_____

_____

DATE: / /

How are you feeling today?

UGH   OK   GOOD   AWESOME

How did you sleep last night?

_____

Breakfast   TIME: _____

FOOD: _____

_____

_____

DRINKS: _____

Lunch   TIME: _____

FOOD: _____

_____

_____

DRINKS: _____

Dinner   TIME: _____

FOOD: _____

_____

_____

DRINKS: _____

Snacks/Other   TIME(S): _____

_____

_____

Supplements/Medications (if applicable)

_____

How many servings of vegetables did you eat today? _____

Exercise

_____

Mindfulness practice

_____

List three things you are grateful for:

1. _____

2. _____

3. _____

What went well today?

_____

_____

_____

LET IT OUT

_____

_____

_____

_____

_____

DATE: / /

How are you feeling today?

UGH   OK   GOOD   AWESOME

How did you sleep last night?

_____

Breakfast   TIME: _____

FOOD: _____

_____

_____

DRINKS: _____

Lunch   TIME: _____

FOOD: _____

_____

_____

DRINKS: _____

Dinner   TIME: _____

FOOD: _____

_____

_____

DRINKS: _____

Snacks/Other   TIME(S): _____

_____

_____

Supplements/Medications (if applicable)

_____

How many servings of vegetables did you eat today? _____

Exercise

_____

Mindfulness practice

_____

List three things you are grateful for:

1. _____

2. _____

3. _____

What went well today?

_____

_____

_____

LET IT OUT

_____

_____

_____

_____

_____

DATE: / /

How are you feeling today?

UGH   OK   GOOD   AWESOME

How did you sleep last night?

_____

Breakfast   TIME: _____

FOOD: _____

_____

_____

DRINKS: _____

Lunch   TIME: _____

FOOD: _____

_____

_____

DRINKS: _____

Dinner   TIME: _____

FOOD: _____

_____

_____

DRINKS: _____

Snacks/Other   TIME(S): _____

_____

_____

Supplements/Medications (if applicable)

_____

How many servings of vegetables did you eat today? ——————————

Exercise

_____

Mindfulness practice

_____

List three things you are grateful for:

1. _____

2. _____

3. _____

What went well today?

_____

_____

_____

LET IT OUT

_____

_____

_____

_____

_____

DATE: /   /

How are you feeling today?

UGH   OK   GOOD   AWESOME

How did you sleep last night?

_____

Breakfast   TIME: _____

FOOD: _____

_____

_____

DRINKS: _____

Lunch   TIME: _____

FOOD: _____

_____

_____

DRINKS: _____

Dinner   TIME: _____

FOOD: _____

_____

_____

DRINKS: _____

Snacks/Other   TIME(S): _____

_____

_____

Supplements/Medications (if applicable)

_____

How many servings of vegetables did you eat today? _____

Exercise

_____

Mindfulness practice

_____

List three things you are grateful for:

1. _____

2. _____

3. _____

What went well today?

_____

_____

_____

LET IT OUT

_____

_____

_____

_____

_____

DATE: / /

How are you feeling today?

UGH   OK   GOOD   AWESOME

How did you sleep last night?

_____

Breakfast   TIME: _____

FOOD: _____

_____

_____

DRINKS: _____

Lunch   TIME: _____

FOOD: _____

_____

_____

DRINKS: _____

Dinner   TIME: _____

FOOD: _____

_____

_____

DRINKS: _____

Snacks/Other   TIME(S): _____

_____

_____

Supplements/Medications (if applicable)

_____

How many servings of vegetables did you eat today? ————————————

Exercise

_____

Mindfulness practice

_____

List three things you are grateful for:

1. _____

2. _____

3. _____

What went well today?

_____

_____

_____

LET IT OUT

_____

_____

_____

_____

_____

DATE: /   /

How are you feeling today?

UGH   OK   GOOD   AWESOME

How did you sleep last night?

_____

Breakfast   TIME: _____

FOOD: _____

_____

_____

DRINKS: _____

Lunch   TIME: _____

FOOD: _____

_____

_____

DRINKS: _____

Dinner   TIME: _____

FOOD: _____

_____

_____

DRINKS: _____

Snacks/Other   TIME(S): _____

_____

_____

Supplements/Medications (if applicable)

_____

How many servings of vegetables did you eat today? ——————————

Exercise

_____

Mindfulness practice

_____

List three things you are grateful for:

1. _____

2. _____

3. _____

What went well today?

_____

_____

_____

LET IT OUT

_____

_____

_____

_____

_____

DATE: / /

How are you feeling today?

UGH   OK   GOOD   AWESOME

How did you sleep last night?

_____

Breakfast   TIME: _____

FOOD: _____

_____

_____

DRINKS: _____

Lunch   TIME: _____

FOOD: _____

_____

_____

DRINKS: _____

Dinner   TIME: _____

FOOD: _____

_____

_____

DRINKS: _____

Snacks/Other   TIME(S): _____

_____

_____

Supplements/Medications (if applicable)

_____

How many servings of vegetables did you eat today? ——————————————

Exercise

_____

Mindfulness practice

_____

List three things you are grateful for:

1. _____

2. _____

3. _____

What went well today?

_____

_____

_____

LET IT OUT

_____

_____

_____

_____

_____

DATE: / /

How are you feeling today?

UGH   OK   GOOD   AWESOME

How did you sleep last night?

_____

Breakfast   TIME: _____

FOOD: _____

_____

_____

DRINKS: _____

Lunch   TIME: _____

FOOD: _____

_____

_____

DRINKS: _____

Dinner   TIME: _____

FOOD: _____

_____

_____

DRINKS: _____

Snacks/Other   TIME(S): _____

_____

_____

Supplements/Medications (if applicable)

_____

How many servings of vegetables did you eat today? —————————————

Exercise

_____

Mindfulness practice

_____

List three things you are grateful for:

1. _____

2. _____

3. _____

What went well today?

_____

_____

_____

LET IT OUT

_____

_____

_____

_____

_____

DATE: /   /

How are you feeling today?

UGH   OK   GOOD   AWESOME

How did you sleep last night?

_____

Breakfast   TIME: _____

FOOD: _____

_____

_____

DRINKS: _____

Lunch   TIME: _____

FOOD: _____

_____

_____

DRINKS: _____

Dinner   TIME: _____

FOOD: _____

_____

_____

DRINKS: _____

Snacks/Other   TIME(S): _____

_____

_____

Supplements/Medications (if applicable)

_____

How many servings of vegetables did you eat today? ———————————

Exercise

_____

Mindfulness practice

_____

List three things you are grateful for:

1. _____

2. _____

3. _____

What went well today?

_____

_____

_____

LET IT OUT

_____

_____

_____

_____

_____

NOTES

NOTES

NOTES

NOTES

REFERENCES

1. Bandura, A. (2005). "The Primacy of Self-Regulation in Health Promotion." *Applied Psychology* 54(2): 245–254. https://doi.org/10.1111/j.1464-0597.2005.00208.x.

2. Strecher, V. J., B. McEvoy DeVellis, M. H. Becker, and I. M. Rosenstock (1986). "The Role of Self-Efficacy in Achieving Health Behavior Change." *Health Education Quarterly* 13(1): 73–92. https://doi.org/10.1177/109019818601300108.

3. Burke, L. E., J. Wang, and M. A. Sevick (2011). "Self-Monitoring in Weight Loss: A Systematic Review of the Literature." *Journal of the American Dietetic Association* 111(1): 92–102. https://doi.org/10.1016/j.jada.2010.10.008.

4. Baker, R. C., and D. S. Kirschenbaum (1993). "Self-Monitoring May Be Necessary for Successful Weight Control." *Behavior Therapy* 24(3): 377–394. https://doi.org/10.1016/S0005-7894(05)80212-6.

MIA RIGDEN / RASA

Mia Rigden is a Los Angeles–based nutritionist and the founder of RASA, a holistic wellness practice. The California-native is a professionally trained chef and believer that for food to be good for you, it must first be delicious. Mia works with clients globally through her signature whole foods detox, the RASA Challenge, one-on-one coaching programs, wellness consulting, and recipe development. Mia is a graduate of the University of California at Santa Barbara, the International Culinary Institute, and the Institute of Integrative Nutrition, and she has a master's degree in Nutrition and Integrative Health from the Maryland University of Integrative Health. You can find her at @the_rasa_life on Instagram or at therasalife.com.

IN COLLABORATION WITH
WILLA CREATIVE AGENCY

Willa Creative Agency is a team of designers, content creators, and brand strategists based in Venice, California. Willa's female-led team crafts design solutions to launch and grow brands. Willa specializes in branding, packaging, content production, and web design and development. You can find them at @willacreative on Instagram or at willaca.com.

All rights reserved.
Published in the United States by Clarkson Potter/Publishers,
an imprint of Random House, a division of Penguin
Random House LLC, New York.
clarksonpotter.com

CLARKSON POTTER is a trademark and POTTER with colophon
is a registered trademark of Penguin Random House LLC.

Originally self-published in the United States,
in slightly different form, by the author in 2019.

ISBN 978-0-593-13941-7

Printed in China

Book design by Ashley Steen

1 3 5 7 9 10 8 6 4 2

FIRST EDITION